DIP DIET

Discover, Implement, Prevail

Yatendra Kumar Singh 'Manuh'

CONTENTS

INTRODUCTION

Welcome to the transformative journey of the DIP Diet, where discovery, implementation, and prevailing over challenges lead to a healthier and more vibrant you. In this comprehensive guide, we will unravel the intricacies of the DIP Diet, providing you with the tools and knowledge to embark on a life-changing path.

The DIP Diet isn't just a weight-loss program; it's a holistic approach to well-being. Rooted in science and fueled by a passion for sustainable health, this book will guide you through fifteen carefully crafted chapters, each unlocking a new facet of the DIP philosophy.

As you navigate the pages ahead, you'll delve into the science behind the DIP Diet, understand how your body responds to different nutritional approaches, and learn to overcome the hurdles that may arise on your journey. We'll explore the power of nutrition, the importance of mental resilience, and the role of exercise in tandem with the DIP lifestyle.

But this isn't just about the mechanics of the diet; it's about creating a sustainable, enjoyable way of life. From crafting delicious DIP-approved recipes to building a supportive community around you, we'll equip you with the tools to not only reach your goals but to maintain them for a lifetime.

Are you ready to embark on a transformative journey? The DIP Diet awaits, promising not just a change in your body but a revolution in your overall well-being.

CHAPTER 1: UNVEILING THE DIP DIET PHILOSOPHY (CONTINUED)

The Essence of Discovery

At the heart of the DIP Diet lies the concept of discovery. Before embarking on any journey, one must first understand oneself—their habits, preferences, and the intricacies of their relationship with food. In this chapter, we delve into the importance of self-discovery, guiding you through reflective exercises that uncover your motivations, triggers, and long-term health goals.

Understanding the driving force behind your desire for change is pivotal in sustaining your commitment to the DIP Diet. Whether it's achieving a healthier weight, managing specific health conditions, or simply enhancing overall well-being, this journey begins with a deep exploration of your personal landscape.

Implementation Strategies

With newfound self-awareness, we transition into the practicalities of implementing the DIP Diet into your daily life. This section is a roadmap, detailing step-by-step guidelines on how to seamlessly integrate the principles of the DIP Diet into your routine. From grocery shopping tips to meal planning strategies, we leave no stone unturned.

Implementation extends beyond just what's on your plate—it involves creating an environment that fosters success. Learn how to set up your kitchen, optimize your daily schedule, and make informed choices that align with the DIP philosophy. This chapter aims to empower you with the tools needed to make the transition from theory to practice a smooth and rewarding experience.

The Prevailing Spirit

The final component of the DIP Diet philosophy is the prevailing spirit—a mindset that propels you forward, even in the face of challenges. We explore the psychological aspects of embracing change, providing insights into building resilience and cultivating a positive mindset. As you navigate through this chapter, you'll discover how to overcome setbacks, stay motivated, and celebrate small victories along the way.

The journey of discovery and implementation sets the stage for the prevailing spirit to take root. This chapter concludes by emphasizing the symbiotic relationship between understanding oneself, adopting practical strategies, and maintaining the mental fortitude required for lasting success.

As you absorb the wisdom within these pages, remember that the DIP Diet is not just a regimen—it's a transformative lifestyle. Join us on this voyage of self-discovery, practical implementation, and the unwavering spirit that defines the DIP philosophy. Your journey towards a healthier, happier you starts here.

CHAPTER 2: THE SCIENCE BEHIND DIP: UNDERSTANDING THE BODY'S RESPONSE

The Body as a Dynamic System

In the second chapter of our exploration into the DIP Diet, we venture into the intricate science that underpins this transformative approach. Understanding how the body responds to different dietary patterns is fundamental to making informed choices. We begin by unraveling the complexity of the human body as a dynamic system, constantly adapting to the fuel we provide.

Metabolism Unveiled

Dive deep into the mechanisms of metabolism, exploring how the body processes and utilizes nutrients. From the thermic effect of food to the role of hormones, this section provides a comprehensive overview. By grasping the intricacies of metabolism, you gain valuable insights into how the DIP Diet can optimize these processes for sustainable health and vitality.

Nutritional Principles in Action

Building upon the foundation of metabolism, we explore the nutritional principles that guide the DIP Diet. From macronutrient balance to the importance of micronutrients, this chapter offers practical knowledge to inform your food choices. Learn how to create meals that not only support your immediate goals but contribute to long-term well-being.

Adapting to Individual Needs

No two bodies are the same, and this chapter addresses the importance of personalized nutrition. Discover how to tailor the DIP Diet to your unique requirements, taking into account factors such as age, activity level, and specific health conditions. Empowered with this knowledge, you can navigate the dietary landscape with confidence, ensuring the DIP approach aligns seamlessly with your individual needs.

The Role of Gut Health

As we conclude this chapter, we delve into the fascinating realm of gut health. Explore the symbiotic relationship between the gut microbiota and overall well-being. Understand how the DIP Diet supports a thriving gut environment, positively influencing not just digestion but also aspects of immune function and mental health.

In the journey through Chapter 2, you'll gain a profound appreciation for the scientific principles that make the DIP Diet not just a trend but a well-founded lifestyle choice. Armed with this knowledge, you're better equipped to make informed decisions that resonate with your body's intricate design. Join us as we bridge the gap between theory and application, unlocking the secrets of how the DIP Diet harmonizes with the science of the human body.

CHAPTER 3: SETTING THE STAGE: PREPARING FOR YOUR DIP JOURNEY

Building a Foundation for Success

As we embark on Chapter 3, we shift our focus to the crucial phase of preparation. Just as a well-built stage sets the scene for a captivating performance, preparing for your DIP journey lays the groundwork for transformative success. This chapter is your guide to creating an environment that fosters commitment, dedication, and sustainable change.

Assessing Readiness and Setting Goals

Before diving headfirst into the DIP Diet, it's essential to assess your readiness for change. This section provides a toolkit for self-reflection, helping you gauge your current habits, motivations, and potential obstacles. Armed with this awareness, you'll craft realistic and achievable goals that will guide you throughout your DIP journey.

The Importance of Accountability

Accountability is a cornerstone of successful lifestyle change.

Explore strategies to build a support system that keeps you on track, whether through friends, family, or online communities. We'll delve into the power of accountability partners, sharing experiences and challenges to strengthen your resolve and motivation.

Creating a DIP-Friendly Environment

Your surroundings play a pivotal role in shaping your habits. Learn how to transform your home, workplace, and social spaces into supportive environments for the DIP lifestyle. From organizing your kitchen to navigating social gatherings, this section provides practical tips to navigate potential challenges with confidence.

Planning for Success

This chapter culminates in the art of strategic planning. We guide you through the process of developing a personalized roadmap for your DIP journey. From weekly meal prep to scheduling physical activity, each aspect of your routine is considered. By the end of this chapter, you'll possess a comprehensive plan designed to propel you toward your health and wellness goals.

In the realm of the DIP Diet, success is not just about what you do on your plate; it's about the holistic alignment of your environment, mindset, and aspirations. Chapter 3 serves as your compass, directing you toward a prepared, purposeful, and empowered beginning to the transformative journey that lies ahead. Join us as we set the stage for your DIP triumph.

CHAPTER 4: DIVE IN: EXPLORING THE FIRST PHASE OF THE DIP DIET

Initiating Your Transformation

In Chapter 4, we take the plunge into the first phase of the DIP Diet —a phase marked by exploration, adaptation, and the initiation of transformative change. As you dive into this segment of your journey, you'll encounter practical strategies, insightful tips, and a wealth of information designed to ease your transition into the DIP lifestyle.

Understanding Phase One

This section provides a comprehensive overview of the initial phase of the DIP Diet. Explore the specific dietary guidelines, recommended food choices, and the science behind the adjustments your body undergoes during this period. By understanding the principles governing Phase One, you gain clarity on the foundations of your transformation.

Navigating Challenges

No transformative journey is without its challenges, and the

DIP Diet is no exception. Chapter 4 equips you with tools to navigate common hurdles, from cravings to social pressures. Discover effective coping mechanisms and strategies to maintain momentum when faced with obstacles, ensuring that challenges become stepping stones rather than roadblocks.

Celebrating Small Wins

Acknowledging progress, no matter how small, is a crucial aspect of the DIP Diet. This section emphasizes the significance of celebrating your achievements. By recognizing and celebrating the positive changes in your lifestyle, you reinforce your commitment and cultivate a positive mindset, key elements for long-term success.

Listening to Your Body

As you immerse yourself in the first phase, Chapter 4 emphasizes the importance of tuning into your body's signals. Learn how to decipher hunger cues, identify satiety, and adapt the DIP guidelines to your unique needs. This attunement fosters a harmonious relationship with food, laying the groundwork for sustained well-being.

Your journey through the initial phase of the DIP Diet is a pivotal stage in your transformation. Chapter 4 serves as your guide, offering insights, strategies, and encouragement as you explore the beginning of this empowering process. Join us as we navigate the waters of change, celebrating the strides you make toward a healthier, more vibrant you.

CHAPTER 5: NAVIGATING CHALLENGES: OVERCOMING HURDLES IN YOUR DIP TRANSFORMATION

Recognizing and Embracing Challenges

As your DIP journey progresses, Chapter 5 delves into the inevitable challenges that may arise. Rather than viewing these hurdles as setbacks, we explore them as opportunities for growth and learning. Understanding the nature of challenges is the first step towards overcoming them and ensuring a resilient and enduring DIP transformation.

Cravings and Temptations

Cravings are a common companion on any dietary journey, and the DIP Diet is no exception. In this section, we dissect the roots of cravings, offering practical strategies to address them. From mindful eating techniques to incorporating satisfying alternatives, you'll learn how to navigate cravings while staying true to your DIP goals.

Social Pressures and Dining Out

Maintaining your DIP commitment in social settings can be challenging, but it's a crucial skill for long-term success. Chapter 5 provides tips on navigating social pressures, making informed choices when dining out, and communicating your dietary preferences effectively. Empower yourself with the knowledge and confidence to enjoy social occasions while staying true to your DIP principles.

Plateaus and Adjustments

Plateaus are a natural part of any transformative journey. This segment explores the reasons behind plateaus in the DIP Diet and outlines strategies to overcome them. From adjusting your nutrition plan to incorporating new forms of physical activity, you'll discover effective ways to reignite progress and momentum.

The Mind-Body Connection

Recognizing the interconnectedness of mental and physical well-being is crucial on the DIP journey. Chapter 5 explores the mind-body connection, offering mindfulness and stress management techniques. By fostering a balanced mental state, you enhance your ability to navigate challenges, make mindful choices, and ultimately prevail in your DIP transformation.

As you navigate Chapter 5, view challenges not as roadblocks, but as stepping stones on your journey to a healthier, more fulfilled life. This chapter is your guide to developing resilience, building coping strategies, and embracing the transformative power of overcoming hurdles in the DIP Diet. Join us as we equip you with the tools to navigate challenges with grace and determination.

CHAPTER 6: THE POWER OF NUTRITION: CRAFTING YOUR DIP DIET MEAL PLANS

Understanding Nutritional Needs

In the sixth chapter of your DIP journey, we delve into the art and science of crafting personalized meal plans. Understanding your unique nutritional needs is paramount to the success of the DIP Diet. This section guides you through the intricacies of macronutrients, micronutrients, and the optimal balance for your individual goals and health requirements.

Designing Balanced and Varied Meals

Building on nutritional principles, we explore the practical side of meal planning. Discover how to design meals that are not only nutritionally rich but also flavorful and satisfying. From breakfast to dinner, this chapter provides ideas, recipes, and tips to create a diverse menu that aligns with the DIP philosophy.

The Role of Timing and Frequency

Meal timing and frequency play a crucial role in the DIP Diet's effectiveness. This section offers insights into the importance of balanced meal distribution throughout the day. Learn how to optimize nutrient absorption, stabilize energy levels, and support your body's natural rhythm through strategic meal planning.

Adapting the DIP Diet to Your Lifestyle

Flexibility is key to sustaining any dietary approach. Chapter 6 guides you in adapting the DIP Diet to fit seamlessly into your lifestyle. Whether you have a busy schedule, dietary restrictions, or specific preferences, this segment provides strategies to ensure that the DIP Diet becomes a practical and enjoyable part of your daily routine.

Nutritional Strategies for Specific Goals

Whether your DIP goals include weight management, improved energy levels, or addressing specific health concerns, this chapter tailors nutritional strategies to your individual objectives. Explore targeted approaches to enhance your DIP experience and achieve the outcomes that matter most to you.

As you immerse yourself in Chapter 6, you're not just creating meal plans; you're cultivating a sustainable and enjoyable way of nourishing your body. Join us on this culinary exploration, where nutrition meets creativity, and mealtime becomes a cornerstone of your DIP success.

CHAPTER 7: STRENGTHENING THE MIND: MENTAL RESILIENCE IN THE DIP PROCESS

Embracing the Mind-Body Connection

Chapter 7 delves into the powerful interplay between mental and physical well-being. Strengthening the mind is a crucial aspect of the DIP process, influencing your ability to stay committed, overcome challenges, and ultimately prevail in your transformative journey.

Mindfulness and Intuitive Eating

Explore the practice of mindfulness and its application to eating through intuitive eating. Learn to listen to your body's signals, distinguish between physical and emotional hunger, and cultivate a mindful relationship with food. This section provides practical exercises and techniques to enhance your awareness and enjoyment of the eating experience.

Goal Setting and Positive Affirmations

Setting and revisiting your goals is a key motivator in the DIP process. Chapter 7 guides you through effective goal-setting techniques, ensuring your objectives align with your evolving aspirations. Additionally, discover the power of positive affirmations in fostering a resilient mindset, cultivating self-belief, and reinforcing your commitment to the DIP lifestyle.

Stress Management Strategies

In the face of life's challenges, stress management becomes paramount. This section equips you with a toolkit of stress-relief strategies, from relaxation techniques to mindful exercises. By managing stress effectively, you enhance your mental resilience, creating a foundation for sustained success in the DIP journey.

Building a Supportive Mindset

Surrounding yourself with a supportive mindset is instrumental in your DIP transformation. Chapter 7 explores the importance of cultivating a positive environment, both internally and externally. Learn how to foster a mindset that embraces progress over perfection, views setbacks as opportunities for growth, and celebrates the journey rather than just the destination.

As you engage with Chapter 7, recognize that mental resilience is not just a byproduct of the DIP process; it's a skill to be cultivated. Join us in fortifying the connection between your mind and your DIP journey, laying the groundwork for enduring well-being and transformation.

CHAPTER 8: SUSTAINING SUCCESS: LONG-TERM STRATEGIES FOR DIP MASTERY

The Art of Consistency

As we delve into Chapter 8, the focus shifts to sustaining the success you've achieved in your DIP journey. Consistency is key, and this chapter serves as your guide to mastering the art of maintaining positive habits and reaping the long-term benefits of the DIP Diet.

Establishing Lifestyle Routines

Explore the integration of DIP principles into your daily life through the establishment of lifestyle routines. From morning rituals to evening practices, this section provides insights into creating habits that not only support your health goals but also enhance your overall well-being.

Progressive Adjustments

Your journey is dynamic, and so should be your approach. Chapter

8 introduces the concept of progressive adjustments, guiding you on how to evolve your DIP strategies as your body, goals, and lifestyle change. This adaptive mindset is crucial for continued success and growth.

Reflecting on Progress

Reflection is a powerful tool for sustaining success. This segment encourages you to regularly reflect on your journey—celebrating achievements, acknowledging challenges, and assessing how far you've come. By understanding your progress, you empower yourself to make informed decisions for the road ahead.

Integrating Enjoyment into Wellness

Sustained success in the DIP Diet is not just about adherence; it's about enjoying the process. Chapter 8 emphasizes the importance of incorporating joy and pleasure into your wellness journey. Discover how to maintain a positive relationship with food, fitness, and self-care, ensuring that your DIP lifestyle remains fulfilling and sustainable.

In Chapter 8, we transition from the initial phases of discovery and implementation to the mastery of the DIP lifestyle. It's not just about reaching your goals; it's about living a life characterized by vitality, balance, and enduring well-being. Join us as we explore the strategies that will propel you toward sustained success in the DIP Diet.

CHAPTER 9: BEYOND THE SCALE: HOLISTIC HEALTH BENEFITS OF THE DIP LIFESTYLE

Redefining Success

In Chapter 9, our exploration transcends traditional measures of success. Beyond the scale, we delve into the holistic health benefits that extend far beyond physical appearance. Discover how the DIP lifestyle positively impacts various facets of your well-being, fostering a comprehensive sense of health and vitality.

Enhanced Energy and Vitality

Uncover the energy-boosting potential of the DIP lifestyle. From nutrient-dense foods to strategic physical activity, learn how these elements synergize to enhance your vitality and overall energy levels. This section guides you in harnessing the power of the DIP Diet to feel more vibrant and invigorated in your daily life.

Improved Sleep Quality

Quality sleep is a cornerstone of well-being. Explore the connection between the DIP lifestyle and improved sleep hygiene. From establishing bedtime rituals to mindful practices, this chapter provides insights into optimizing your sleep patterns for enhanced rest and recovery.

Mental Clarity and Focus

The benefits of the DIP lifestyle extend beyond the body to encompass the mind. Discover how nutrition, mindfulness, and lifestyle choices influence mental clarity and focus. This section offers practical strategies to enhance cognitive function, supporting your overall mental well-being.

Embracing Emotional Wellness

Emotional wellness is an integral part of the DIP journey. Chapter 9 explores the connection between the foods you consume and your emotional state. Learn how the DIP lifestyle fosters emotional resilience and discover techniques to navigate stress, promote joy, and cultivate emotional well-being.

As we journey into Chapter 9, redefine your understanding of success in the DIP Diet. It's not just about external transformations but about cultivating a holistic sense of well-being that radiates from within. Join us as we explore the profound, multifaceted benefits that the DIP lifestyle brings to every aspect of your health and vitality.

CHAPTER 10: DIP AND EXERCISE: FINDING THE PERFECT BALANCE

The Synergy of Diet and Exercise

In Chapter 10, we explore the dynamic relationship between the DIP Diet and exercise, recognizing that a holistic approach to well-being involves both nutritional choices and physical activity. This chapter is your guide to finding the perfect balance, ensuring that your exercise routine complements and enhances the benefits of the DIP lifestyle.

Tailoring Exercise to Your Goals

Whether your fitness goals include weight management, strength building, or overall cardiovascular health, this section provides insights into tailoring your exercise routine to align with your objectives. Discover how different forms of exercise synergize with the principles of the DIP Diet to maximize your health outcomes.

Incorporating Movement into Daily Life

Exercise is not confined to the gym; it's a dynamic part of

daily life. Chapter 10 explores ways to incorporate movement seamlessly into your routine, from active commuting to simple at-home exercises. By integrating physical activity into your daily life, you enhance the sustainability of your fitness journey.

Finding Joy in Movement

The DIP lifestyle emphasizes the enjoyment of the wellness journey, and this applies to exercise as well. Discover how to find joy in movement, selecting activities that resonate with your interests and preferences. Whether it's dancing, hiking, or practicing yoga, this chapter encourages you to embrace activities that bring fulfillment and satisfaction.

Recovery and Restorative Practices

Recognizing the importance of recovery is integral to a balanced fitness routine. Chapter 10 explores restorative practices, from stretching and yoga to mindful breathing exercises. By prioritizing recovery, you optimize the benefits of your exercise routine and contribute to the overall well-being fostered by the DIP lifestyle.

As you navigate Chapter 10, strike a harmonious balance between the nourishment provided by the DIP Diet and the invigoration brought by exercise. Join us in discovering how the synergy of diet and exercise propels you towards a state of vibrant health, where movement becomes not just a routine but an integral part of your joyful, DIP-inspired lifestyle.

CHAPTER 11: CULINARY CREATIVITY: DELICIOUS RECIPES FOR DIP SUCCESS

Elevating Your Culinary Experience

In Chapter 11, we venture into the realm of culinary creativity, transforming your DIP Diet into a delightful gastronomic adventure. This chapter serves as your culinary guide, providing a diverse array of delicious recipes that not only align with DIP principles but also elevate your eating experience.

Nutrient-Dense and Flavorful Meals

Discover the art of crafting meals that are both nutrient-dense and bursting with flavor. From vibrant salads to hearty mains, each recipe is a celebration of wholesome ingredients, carefully balanced to ensure you not only meet your nutritional needs but also savor every bite.

Exploring DIP-Friendly Cuisines

Embark on a global culinary journey as we explore DIP-friendly adaptations of various cuisines. From Mediterranean delights to Asian-inspired dishes, this section introduces you to the rich tapestry of flavors that can be seamlessly integrated into the DIP lifestyle.

Quick and Convenient Options

Recognizing the importance of convenience in our fast-paced lives, Chapter 11 offers quick and easy recipes that fit seamlessly into your busy schedule. These time-efficient options ensure that you can maintain the DIP Diet without compromising on taste or nutrition.

Sweet Indulgences with a Healthy Twist

Satisfy your sweet cravings with DIP-friendly desserts that prove healthy eating can be synonymous with indulgence. Discover innovative ways to incorporate natural sweeteners, wholesome ingredients, and creative flavors into your dessert repertoire.

As you explore the culinary wonders of Chapter 11, you'll not only expand your recipe repertoire but also cultivate a newfound appreciation for the joy of nourishing your body. Join us in the kitchen as we blend the art of culinary creativity with the science of the DIP Diet, proving that healthy eating is not just a necessity but a delightful experience.

CHAPTER 12: SOCIAL SUPPORT: BUILDING A DIP COMMUNITY AROUND YOU

The Power of Connection

In Chapter 12, we explore the impact of social support on your DIP journey. Building a supportive community around you is a key element in sustaining motivation, overcoming challenges, and celebrating successes. This chapter delves into the power of connection and offers strategies for fostering a DIP community.

Engaging with Like-Minded Individuals

Connect with individuals who share similar goals and values. Whether through local meet-ups, online forums, or social media groups, discover the joy of engaging with like-minded people. Share experiences, swap recipes, and draw inspiration from the collective wisdom of a community united by the DIP lifestyle.

Family and Friends as Allies

Navigate the dynamics of family and friends, transforming them into allies on your DIP journey. Chapter 12 provides insights into effective communication, setting boundaries, and enlisting the support of those closest to you. Learn to create an environment that encourages shared goals and mutual encouragement.

Group Activities and Challenges

Discover the motivational power of group activities and challenges. From fitness classes to cooking clubs, this section explores ways to turn your DIP journey into a shared adventure. By participating in group challenges, you not only stay accountable but also foster a sense of camaraderie and friendly competition.

Celebrating Milestones Together

Celebrate your DIP achievements with your community. From small victories to significant milestones, Chapter 12 encourages the practice of acknowledging and applauding each other's successes. This shared celebration reinforces the collective strength of your DIP community.

As you delve into Chapter 12, recognize that your DIP journey doesn't have to be a solo endeavor. Embrace the support of a community that understands and uplifts you, turning your individual transformation into a shared, empowering experience. Join us in exploring the transformative power of social support within the context of the DIP lifestyle.

CHAPTER 13: OVERCOMING PLATEAUS: STRATEGIES FOR CONTINUOUS PROGRESS

Understanding Plateaus

In Chapter 13, we address a common challenge on any wellness journey—the plateau. Explore the science behind plateaus in the context of the DIP Diet and gain insights into why they occur. This chapter serves as your guide to overcoming plateaus and ensuring continuous progress towards your health and well-being goals.

Assessing and Adjusting

Learn how to assess your current situation, identify signs of a plateau, and differentiate between temporary fluctuations and a sustained plateau. Chapter 13 provides strategies for making informed adjustments to your DIP lifestyle, ensuring that you break through plateaus and continue on your transformative path.

Introducing Variety

Plateaus can often be broken by introducing variety into your routine. This section explores the importance of diversifying your meals, exercise routines, and even mindfulness practices. Discover how incorporating new elements can reinvigorate your body and mind, propelling you past stagnant points in your DIP journey.

Periodization Techniques

Explore the concept of periodization, a strategic approach to managing your DIP lifestyle in cycles. Chapter 13 guides you through the implementation of different phases, each designed to challenge your body in unique ways and prevent stagnation. Learn how to structure your DIP journey for sustained progress.

Monitoring and Adjusting Goals

Your goals are dynamic, just like your journey. This chapter emphasizes the importance of regularly monitoring and adjusting your goals. By aligning your aspirations with your current circumstances, you ensure that your DIP experience remains both challenging and rewarding.

As you navigate through Chapter 13, recognize plateaus not as roadblocks but as opportunities for growth and refinement. Join us in exploring strategies that not only break through stagnant points but also contribute to the continuous evolution of your DIP lifestyle.

CHAPTER 14: CELEBRATING MILESTONES: REFLECTING ON YOUR DIP ACHIEVEMENTS

The Significance of Milestones

As we enter Chapter 14, the focus shifts to celebrating the milestones achieved on your DIP journey. Recognizing and celebrating successes, both big and small, is a vital component of maintaining motivation and sustaining long-term commitment. This chapter guides you through the art of reflection and celebration.

Setting Milestones Effectively

Learn how to set realistic and meaningful milestones that align with your overall DIP goals. Chapter 14 explores the importance of breaking down your journey into manageable steps, making your progress measurable and your achievements attainable. By setting effective milestones, you create a roadmap for success.

Reflecting on Progress

Take a moment to reflect on how far you've come. This section encourages mindful reflection, acknowledging the challenges overcome, the habits formed, and the positive changes experienced. By appreciating your journey, you reinforce your commitment to the DIP lifestyle.

Cultivating a Positive Mindset

Celebrate milestones with a positive mindset. Chapter 14 explores the transformative power of positivity, encouraging you to focus on the progress made rather than dwelling on setbacks. By cultivating a positive mindset, you create a foundation for continued success and resilience.

Sharing Success Stories

Connect with the broader DIP community by sharing your success stories. Whether through social media, support groups, or local meet-ups, this section explores the impact of sharing your journey. By inspiring others, you contribute to the collective motivation and reinforce your own commitment to the DIP lifestyle.

As you engage with Chapter 14, embrace the art of celebration and reflection. Your DIP journey is a series of achievements and transformations, each deserving recognition. Join us in exploring the significance of milestones and celebrating the remarkable progress you've made towards a healthier, happier you.

CHAPTER 15: FOREVER DIP: EMBRACING A LIFELONG COMMITMENT TO WELLNESS

A Lifestyle, Not a Destination

As we conclude your transformative journey with Chapter 15, it's time to embrace the concept of "Forever DIP." The DIP lifestyle is not a temporary fix but a commitment to lifelong wellness. This chapter explores the strategies, mindset, and practices that will support you in maintaining the benefits of the DIP Diet for the long term.

Reinforcing Habits

Reflect on the habits cultivated throughout your DIP journey and discover how to reinforce them for lasting success. This section provides insights into habit formation, habit stacking, and creating an environment that supports your continued commitment to the DIP lifestyle.

Adapting to Life Changes

Life is dynamic, and so should be your approach to wellness. Chapter 15 guides you through the process of adapting the DIP lifestyle to changing circumstances, whether it's shifts in work, family dynamics, or personal goals. By embracing flexibility, you ensure that the DIP Diet remains a sustainable and integral part of your life.

Continued Learning and Growth

Explore the importance of continued learning on your wellness journey. This chapter encourages you to stay informed about nutrition, fitness trends, and evolving health practices. By cultivating a mindset of growth, you empower yourself to make informed choices that align with your evolving understanding of well-being.

Fostering a Supportive Community

Chapter 15 reinforces the significance of a supportive community. Whether you maintain connections with your initial DIP community or create new circles, having a network that shares your commitment to wellness provides ongoing encouragement and inspiration.

As you conclude your journey with Chapter 15, embrace the concept of "Forever DIP" as a philosophy that transcends diets and quick fixes. Your commitment to lifelong wellness is a testament to the transformative power of the DIP lifestyle. Congratulations on reaching this milestone, and may your journey continue to be a source of inspiration and well-being.

ACKNOWLEDGEMENT

Writing a comprehensive book is a journey filled with inspiration, support, and collaboration. As the author of "DIP Diet: Nourishing the Body, Transforming the Lifestyle," I extend my heartfelt gratitude to those whose contributions and encouragement have been instrumental in bringing this work to fruition.

I would like to express my deepest thanks to the team at AIPRM Corp. for providing the initial prompt that sparked the creation of this book. Your innovative approach to content generation has been the catalyst for a transformative journey in the realm of wellness.

To the individuals who shared their insights, experiences, and expertise in the fields of nutrition, fitness, and mindfulness – your wisdom has enriched the content of this book and added valuable layers to the DIP philosophy.

A special acknowledgment goes to the dedicated community members who actively engaged in discussions, shared personal stories, and offered support throughout the writing process. Your enthusiasm and commitment to the DIP lifestyle have been a continuous source of motivation.

I extend my gratitude to friends and family whose unwavering support and understanding allowed me the time and space to delve into the intricacies of the DIP Diet, turning it from concept to reality.

Last but not least, a sincere thank you to the readers who embark on this journey. Your curiosity, commitment to well-being, and openness to transformation fuel the purpose of this book.

May the pages of "DIP Diet: Nourishing the Body, Transforming the Lifestyle" inspire positive changes in your life and contribute to your ongoing journey of health and happiness.

With gratitude,

Yatendra Kumar Singh 'Manuh'
Author

www.ingramcontent.com/pod-product-compliance
Lightning Source LLC
Chambersburg PA
CBHW060902260726
48661CB00008B/3415